A DEEP DIVE INTO YOGA: A QUICK READ FOR BEGINNERS

BY: CHRIS MATTHERS

TABLE OF CONTENTS

WHAT IS YOGA?

Yoga means "union"; the union of body, mind, and spirit and the union between the being and the cosmic spirit of creation, the unity of all things. This union also applies to our relationship with ourselves, others, and the world around us. Since ancient times, it has been developed in India to help man find well-being, happiness, and unity in his body and soul.

As a pleasant, refreshing, and at the same time relaxing practice, Yoga brings everyone their right rhythm (Yama and Nyama) to connect to relaxation and well-being, harmony, and inner peace, while increasing flexibility and strength (vitality) on the physical, energetic, and mental levels. Letting go and tone, inner listening, and availability allow you to live more harmoniously and holistically.

With kindness and precision, Yoga offers physical postures (asana), punctuated by the breath (pranayama); it brings back to serious attention (pratyahara) and concentration (Dharana); it leads, progressively, to a meditative state (dhyana), allowing relaxation, stability, and joy. As the practice progresses, balance and harmony settle in and around oneself (fluidity between oneself and the world); well-being develops, creativity awakens, and consciousness rises.

Yoga is not a religion but a philosophy and practice based on the principles of the wisdom of life applicable to all. Yoga can lead you to relaxation, balance, focus, and self-control. It will awaken you to a renewed feeling of harmony, allowing you to find yourself little by little. It will also help you access inner peace, discover your hidden potential, improve your health, tone your muscles and organs, decrease nervous tension, reduce your weight, and strengthen your bones.

Yoga is a control of body and brain that incorporates a wide assortment of activities and methods. The strategies utilized utilize actual stances (called asanas), breathing practices (pranayama), and reflection, just as profound unwinding (yoga Nidra). It is an essentially practical system that can enormously help people in everyday life and explore the deeper aspects of life. It offers answers to modern man's problems in the face of stress and difficulty to manage life situations. Yoga is compared to gentle gymnastics, an effective way despite everything to obtain health and well-being.

ORIGIN OF YOGA

Yoga is a school of Indian philosophy that was practiced in India from the 3rd millennium BC. Although of Eastern origin, it has been very well integrated and put into practice in the West, whether in its original form or an adapted form. To go even further, you should know that Yoga is one of India's six great philosophical systems. It is found in some texts under the name of "darsana," meaning "to look at the world." It made its appearance in the 7th century BC in certain writings.

India is the original land of Yoga. Its history is closely linked to that of Indian civilization. It is a discipline developed since ancient times to help human beings go through suffering and find unity and joy in their body and soul. Yoga is part of one of the six major philosophical systems of India. It is a darsana, a term that means to look at the world.

Yoga then appears in all the spiritual pieces of literature of India, where it always designates forms of discipline that unite body and mind, man and the universe, the human and the divine. Anything that can be "joined" to provide a state of happiness, fullness, or liberation, making complementary what may seem to be opposed (day and night, moon and sun, etc.).

Yoga has diversified according to the contexts in which it is practiced. We can distinguish five main paths. First of all, it accompanies the human being in his daily life by helping him to lay down the principles of the "right action," or "disinterested": this is karma-yoga, or "yoga of action." It is also found associated with religious and spiritual currents, within Hinduism or Buddhism, where it allows one to get closer to the divinity: it is bhakti-yoga or "yoga of devotion." It refines the most subtle intelligence, that of realities considered to be beyond the natural, and is then called jnâna-yoga, or "yoga of knowledge." Specific research concerning the body, the breath, and energies has been developed and has given us the most famous and practiced form of Yoga of the West, hatha-yoga. The fifth way brings together the four preceding ones; it is raja-yoga, the royal way all human beings' possibilities are united and explored.

Today, the many traditions of Yoga which have continued to evolve over the generations, continue to be very much alive in India. Some teachers are true spiritual masters; others are simply yoga teachers, with no other ambition than to offer psycho-bodily hygiene adapted to current life. Often less practiced than one thinks by the Indians, Yoga is developing more and more, sometimes as gymnastics, which has always been part of their culture, at school in particular, or as a preventive activity in any form of illness. But it should be emphasized that many do it from a spiritual perspective, to "free themselves" from the conditioning of existence.

THE STAGES OF YOGA

The study of the eight limbs of Yoga adds to the purification of the body, the mind, and the intellect; the flame of knowledge is kept alight, and discernment is awakened. Here are the eight members:

1. Yama

Conduct towards others or social discipline. This includes:

- Non-violence (cultivating love),
- Sincerity (truth, authenticity in thought, word, and deed),
- Non-lust (being satisfied with what is right for you),
- Moderation (preserve vitality)
- Non-greed (freeing oneself from the desire to possess).

These principles apply at all times, places, times, occasions, and these qualities lead to purity.

2. Niyama

Self-discipline or personal discipline, physical and mental:

- Cleanliness (hygiene, healthy food),

- Contentment (serene acceptance of the present moment),
- Austerity (the assiduous practice of purity of thought, word, and action),
- Self-study (self-knowledge and study of the mysteries of the universe),
- Devotion (having confidence and faith, relying on the higher).

These rules should apply to everyone, whether one follows the path of Yoga or not.

3. Asana Postures

The practice of Yoga is within the outermost aspect of the personality: the physical body. Asanas help us keep the body healthy by releasing the tension, massaging internal organs, improving their function, and providing more flexibility to the spine, muscles, and joints.

Asana means to hold the body in a given posture with the idea that the Whole is in itself. The pose must be held firmly to establish unity in oneself. The conquest of the asana occurs when the effort ceases and stability set in. Stability brings about a state of bliss. An asana held in this state is not performed by the physical or physiological body but by the inner self. In this state of the body, the dualities disappear, and the union of body, mind, and soul is achieved. The asana is the perfect firmness of the body, the intelligence's stability, and the spirit's benevolence.

4. Pranayama Breath control

Breathing techniques are important not only for the oxygen supply they provide to the body (all organs and cells) and the lungs' strengthening. They also directly affect the brain and our emotions, balancing the nervous system and bringing us in contact with more subtle energies (like solar, lunar, and Kundalini energy) and other aspects of our being.

Prana is the air, the breath, the life energy. Ayama means its expansion in length, breadth, and volume. Making the breath more conscious, deep, and more subtle will help nourish the posture, stabilize the mind, and calm the whole nervous system. The breath and the reason being linked, a calm breath induces a quiet mind. Several pranayama techniques are proposed using inspiration, expiration, suspension, retention.

5. Pratyahara (The discipline of the senses)

The five sense organs come into contact with the outside world at the instigation of the mind. This extraversion, caused by their desire for worldly objects, must be restrained and directed inward. It is the process of acquiring knowledge of self or cognition: object, the organ of senses, mind, and soul combine and form knowledge. Diverting the mind from the sense organs by bringing them inward is pratyahara.

6. Dharana Concentration

Concentration is defined as the convergence of all the senses on the individual soul. The mind wanders in different directions under the influence of the five senses or subtle qualities: smell, taste, sight, touch, sound. When the mind, the intellect, and the ego are focused on the self, within it is concentration. When this practice is mastered, the way is opened for meditation.

For the two principles above (The principle of senses and concentration), various tools / supports help us to walk: control and direct the senses by paying attention to the movement of the breath (breathing), maintaining our gaze on the flame of a candle, recitation of a mantra, maintaining a comfortable posture, etc.

7. Dyana Meditation

When concentration is prolonged and is kept attentive, it becomes a meditation without a limit of time or space. Nothing disturbs the mediator; thus, the body, the breath, the mind, the intellect, and the ego lose all individual existence and merge into the only state of being. This fusion of the individual soul with the universal soul is meditation.

8. Samadhi 8th and last step of Yoga: Self-realization

At this stage, the individual identity is immersed outwardly and inwardly in meditation. The mediator, the act of meditating, and the object of meditation all lose their characteristics and merge into a single view of the entire cosmos—knowledge of supreme happiness, free from pleasure, pain, or suffering.

Methods and Types of Yoga

There are so many types of Yoga there, whether you want a more physically demanding class or a comfortable, relaxing, meditative class.

With each style somewhat not quite the same as the others, you'll find varieties depending on the educator. Giving a couple of styles and instructors an attempt prior to settling on your favorite will upgrade your general yoga experience and challenge you to break out of your usual range of familiarity.

Here are the major types of Yoga:

1. HATHA YOGA: THE CLASSIC

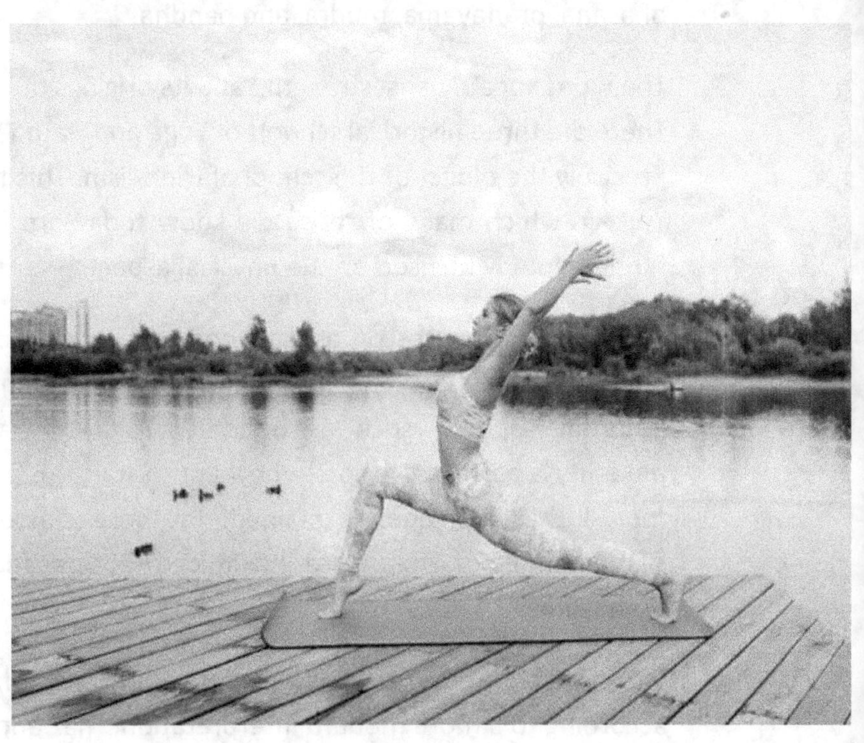

Hatha yoga is an umbrella term that encompasses most Yoga time styles; several Hatha Yoga schools have developed, introducing their sequences and combinations of asana, pranayama, mudra, and bandha.

The word Yoga means 'strength,' and its origin is uncertain. There are three historical schools of Yoga and Hatha Yoga is precisely the oldest of the school of Hinduism. This type of Yoga in which many of those we know today are framed fundamentally focused on the physical aspect.

This practice focuses on asanas, postures, pranayama, or breathing, instead of other types of Yoga at dealing with different aspects, such as Buddhist Yoga tantra. This modality is perfect for those who want to start this practice for all that has been explained. In these classes, the fundamentals of Yoga were introduced, both asanas and pranayama.

The word Hatha means "energetic" or "willful," but according to a more modern interpretation, "ha" and "the" represent the sun and the moon. The soul is viewed as like the sun, failing to change in splendor. The moon resembles our mind, which has vacillations and stages. Through the act of Hatha Yoga, we try to join this double energy to help bring harmony to mind and body.

Hatha yoga permits you to work both body and mind. While improving your adaptability and working on your bodybuilding, this type of Yoga will empower you to abandon your day-by-day stresses unwind.

2.   ASHTANGA YOGA: THE DYNAMIC

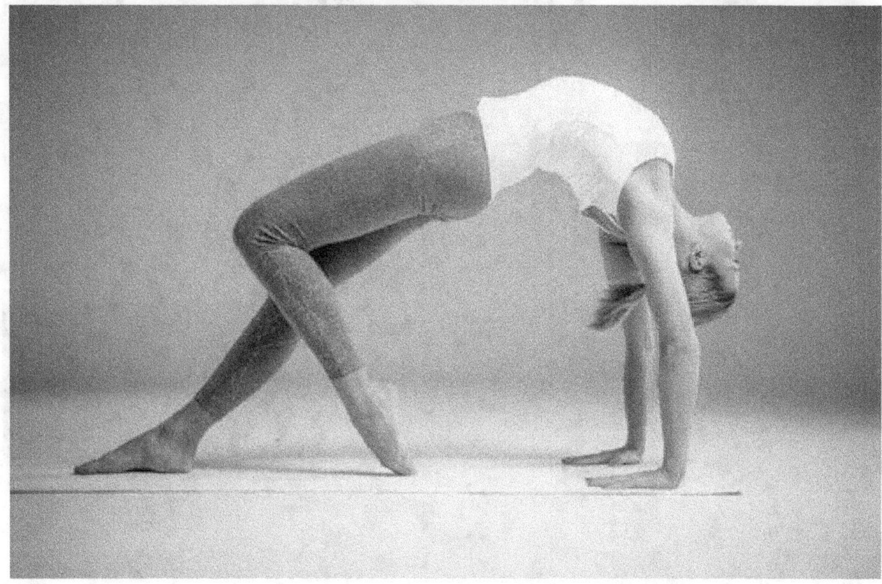

The synchronization of the breath with the movements is the basis of this modality. This is possibly one of the most physical styles along with vinyasa, which is also related to. Its sequences' physical effort detoxifies the body and helps blood circulation, and strengthens the upper body. This form of Yoga involves a rapid series of positions that combine breathing and action. ASHTANGA yoga strengthens the muscles and improves your flexibility.

3. KUNDALINI YOGA: THE STABLE

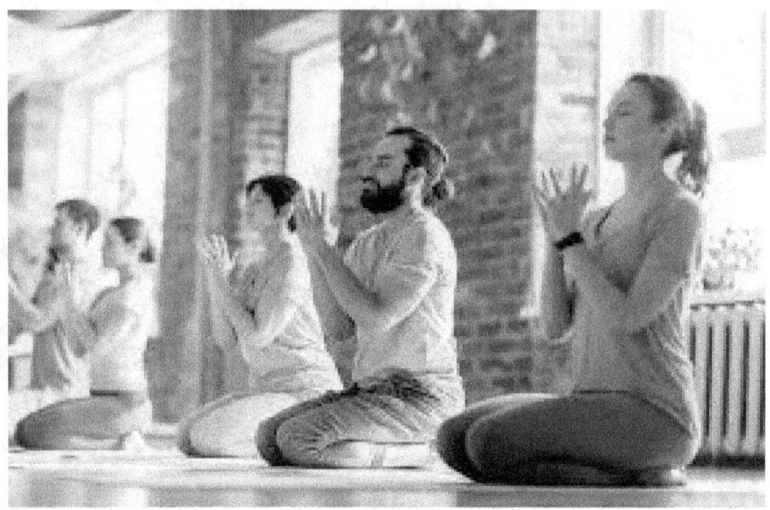

This type of Yoga an addition to postures and breathing incorporates meditation techniques and mantras. It is based on the repetition of a sequence and continuous breathing to put in motion the energy from the first to the last chakra (each of the human body's energy centers that govern organic, psychic, and emotional functions). It is based on various paths of Yoga not only Hatha but also has physical and spiritual components. This is a good practice for those who have high-stress levels and can benefit from meditative ways to combat their symptoms.

It is also known under the name of "yoga of consciousness" because it is Yoga characterized by a vital spiritual component. The postures it promotes, combined with breathing exercises (pranayama) and mantras, seek to balance the chakras to prevent physical and emotional illness. It is an extremely fluid type of Yoga that moderate physical activity.

Kundalini is made up of kriyas, repetitive exercises combined with intense breathing (as if you were breathing fire); this practice can be physically demanding and energizing. Through movement, breathing, and sounds (chanting), you will begin to stimulate and release untapped energy in your spine and through your energy centers, also called chakras.

Classes are usually one hour or longer. The Kundalini is for people who are already used to the world of Yoga between stable postures, choreography, and breathing exercises; the goal is above all to focus the session around the spine. Its benefits are quite intimate; this kind of Yoga allows you to develop knowledge of yourself and your body.

4.   YIN YOGA

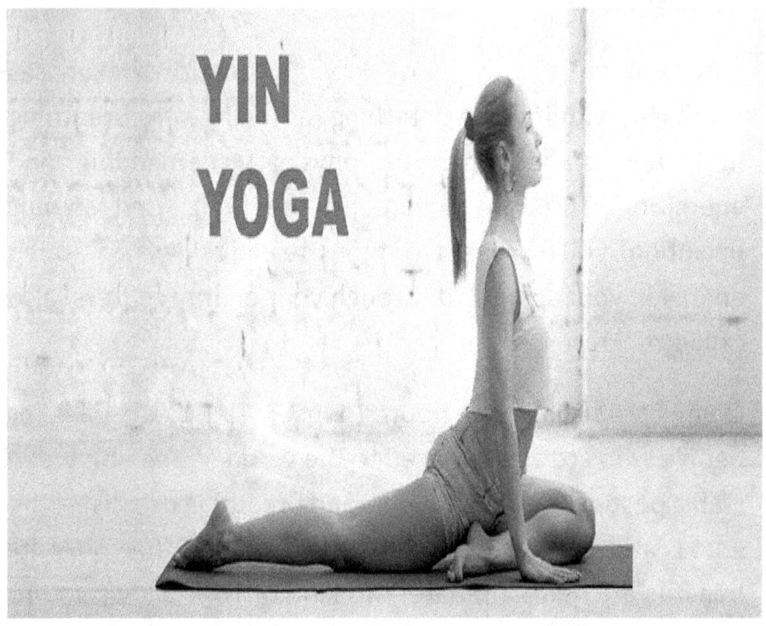

This is one of the slower varieties of Yoga that emphasizes the joints of the body and the skin's deeper tissues. Its meditative incentive means that it can also help combat anxiety and stress as well as increase relaxation. This type of Yoga is also great for beginners.

5. VINYASA YOGA: THE DANCING

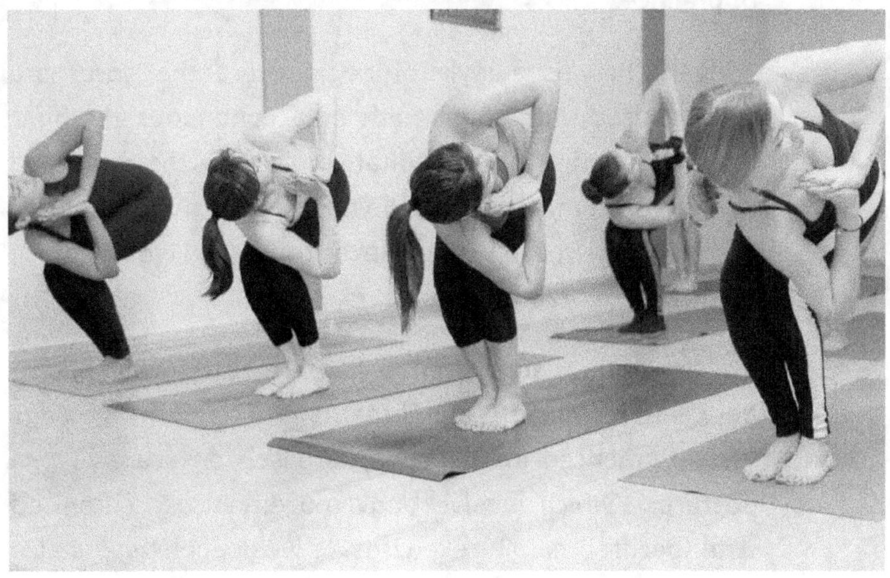

This word could be translated as 'align concretely.' Hatha derived this type of Yoga, intending to synchronize breathing and movement to create a certain fluidity. It is an adaptation of the ASHTANGA that has been practiced since the eighties, leading to other variants such as power yoga. This style is perfect for those who want to strengthen their muscles and learn new postures and a different sequence in each class.

Vinyasa yoga is also called "flow yoga" or "vinyasa flow." It is an incredibly common style. It was adapted from the more regimented ASHTANGA practice a couple of decades ago. The word "vinyasa" translates to "place in a special way," which is often interpreted as linking breath and movement. You'll often see terms like slow, dynamic, or mindful paired with vinyasa or flow to indicate the intensity of practice.

Vinyasa flow is a style of Yoga where the poses are synchronized with the breath in a continuous rhythmic flow. The flow can be meditative, calming the mind and nervous system, even though you're moving. Vinyasa yoga is suitable for those who've never tried Yoga well as those who've been practicing for years.

Vinyasa is the name given in Sanskrit to the relationship between movement and breathing. This form of Yoga widely practiced in the West, is based on asanas (yoga postures), which involve body movements synchronized with specific breathing exercises. As we deepen the practice of this Yoga, the postures' level of difficulty increases, even if the sessions always end with relaxation exercises.

This form of Yoga is based on the sequence of choreographies and stable postures. You could almost believe in a dance class. While performing vinyasa yoga, you will discover an unparalleled synergy between breathing and bodybuilding, and you will improve your balance and flexibility.

6. BIKRAM YOGA: L'INTENSE

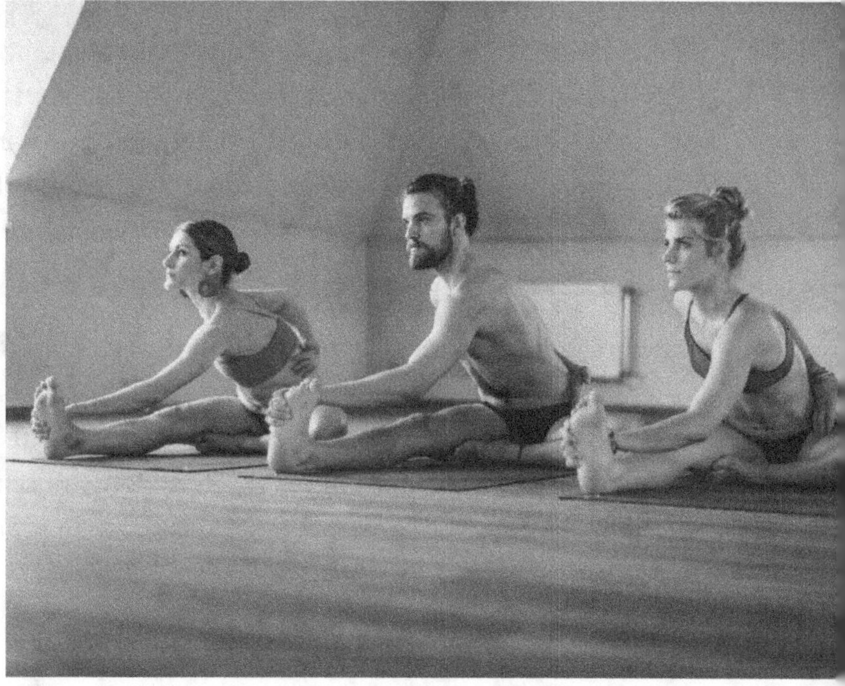

The yogi Bikram Chourdy was the inventor of this modality, in which a sequence of asanas from the Hatha is repeated in a room at 40 °C. In addition to the benefits of Yoga, it can also help vasodilation and eliminate toxins from the body, although this last benefit has not been scientifically proven. It includes a variety of 26 postures combined with breathing exercises in which you sweat a lot, making it perfect for flushing out toxins and losing weight. Usually, the sessions last 90 minutes and can involve an exercise equivalent to 20 minutes of running.

When you walk into a Bikram yoga studio, the first thing you will notice is the warmth. Each studio is heated to approx.

105 degrees (° F) and has a humidity of 40 percent. During the 90-minute class, you will practice a set of 26 poses, such as the balancing stick and the grasshopper pose and two breathing exercises that, according to founder Bikram Choudhury, systematically circulate oxygenated blood throughout the body.

There are 26 postures for the best possible stretch. To intensify the benefits, some have adopted the habit of doing 40 of these postures in a room heated to 40 °C. The heat helps to stress the stretching of tendons, muscles, and ligaments. You will come out more relaxed than ever.

7. YOGA NIDRA: L'INTERIORISÉ

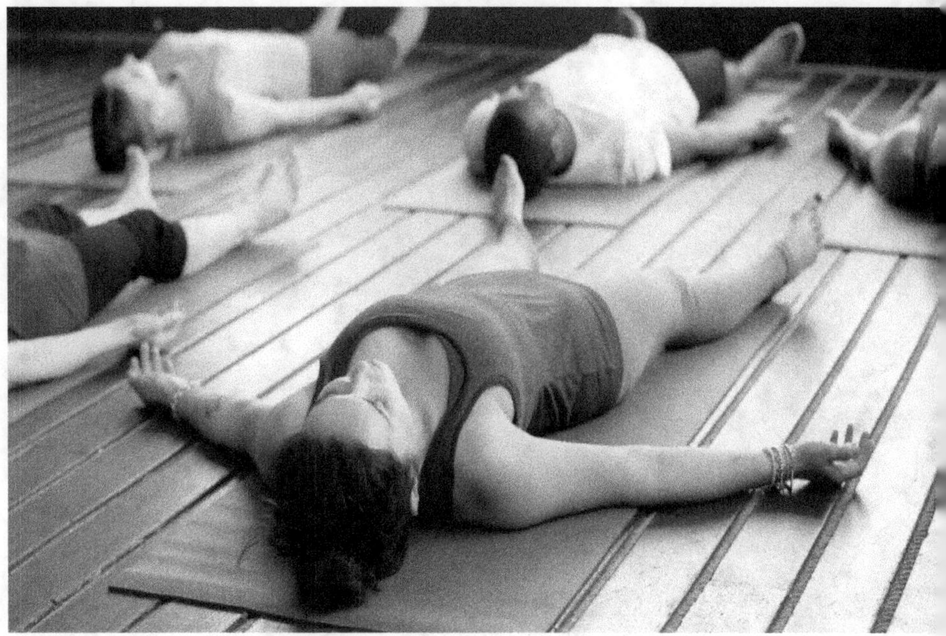

Yoga Nidra involves focusing everything on meditation so that our consciousness takes control of our body. The mind is in a sort of semi-sleep, and our body is totally under the influence of the mind. While performing this activity, you will get to know your body better than anyone, and you will experience significant relaxation.

8. IYENGAR YOGA

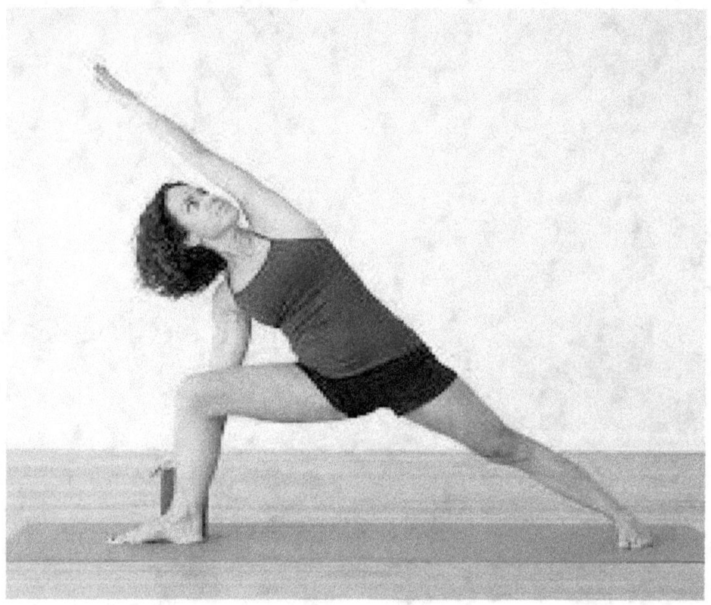

In this modality, the eight stages of Yoga worked, including moral precepts and ethical disciplines, including postures, breathing, and meditation. It is characterized by a sequence in which each pose is held for much longer than in other styles, helping students refine them individually. This Yoga is much slower than others and infers a lot in flexibility, making it ideal for people in rehabilitation for injuries and chronic pain.

Iyengar yoga aims to pay precise attention to our alignment during each posture. You will use various props such as blocks, blankets, straps, folding chairs, and even string walls to find the right alignment for each position. Rather than switching between poses quickly, you will need to hold each pose for a more extended period.

For your first time practicing Iyengar yoga, start with a Level 1 class even if you have done yoga before. This will allow you to learn the fundamentals of this discipline. Classes usually last an hour and a half. Iyengar yoga can be therapeutic for people who are recovering from certain wounds.

Traditional Yoga is revisited to intensify the basic. We focus particularly on the alignment of the body's limbs, which will allow us to follow suitably and quickly the postures. It helps work on your balance, on your blood circulation and concentration.

9. HOT YOGA

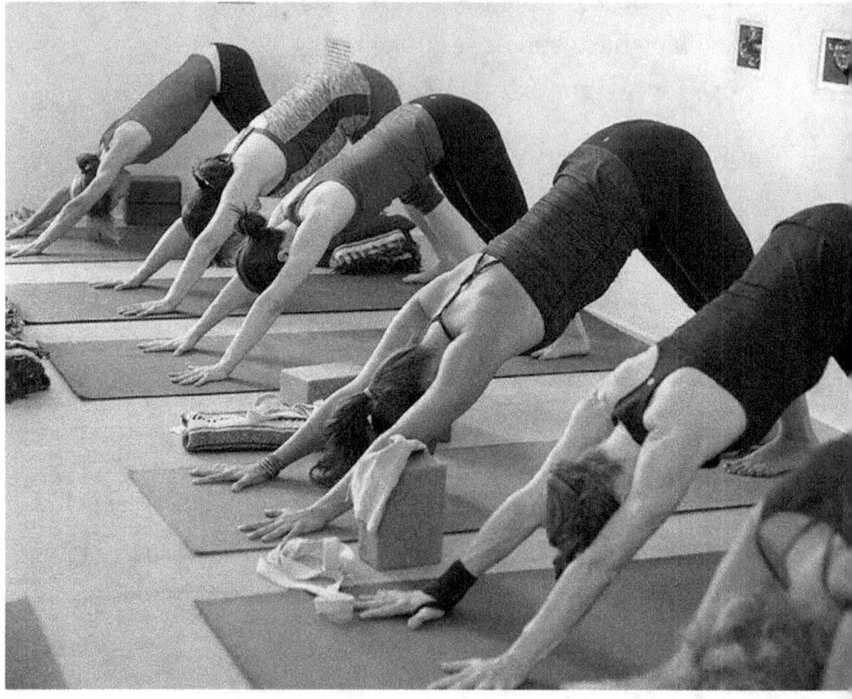

As with the Bikram, be prepared to sweat. Hot Yoga is practiced in a heated room, but the teachers do not follow the Bikram sequences. Instead, teachers are free to vary the series of positions taught during the course.

But beware - while the added heat can help you do more stretched movements, it can be easy to overdo it. Listen to your body, and don't forget to hydrate.

As with Bikram Yoga, Hot Yoga is practiced in a room where the temperature reaches 30 °C. The goal is to perform postures to balance the whole body. Breathing sets the pace for the sequence of different poses, promoting relaxation and control of one's breath.

Hot Yoga is notably recognized for its benefits in terms of relaxation in the neck and back. In addition to strengthening the body's strength and flexibility, Hot Yoga contributes to the release of the hips and shoulders.

10. Restorative Yoga

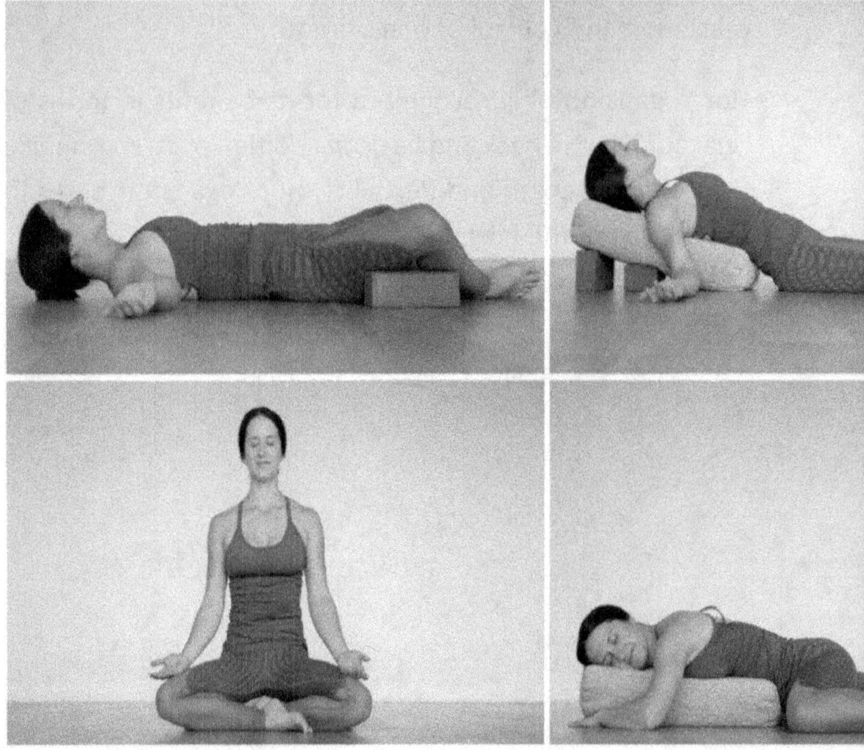

Those who want to get rid of tension can try restorative Yoga which will help muscle relaxation through stretches created by yogi Bellur Krishnamachar Sundararaja Iyengar. Also, within this type of yoga where are passive and active modalities, the first being for static postures in which different accessories such as blocks, ribbons, etc., are used. It is very beneficial for people in physical rehabilitation and can also be useful for pregnant women.

POSES OF YOGA

You may practice Yoga after work or attend a class on the weekends, but doing it as soon as you wake up can change how you feel the rest of the day. Yoga is an excellent practice to start the day, as it puts the body in motion and activates circulation. If you do a few simple poses each morning, your body will wake up, your mind will be more active, and you will feel refreshed.

Yoga is based on three pillars: meditation, breathing, and asanas (postures). It is an activity aimed at harmonizing the body and mind. The practice of Yoga has multiple physical and emotional benefits, including losing weight, maintaining energy, relieving tension and contractures, and improving flexibility and posture.

Many people think that to start Yoga; you have to be super flexible. But really, everyone starts at different points. And usually, everything begins with the first breath. If you remember to breathe, then everything else will fall into place. The following are basic poses for beginners.

1. **Loto (Padmasana)**

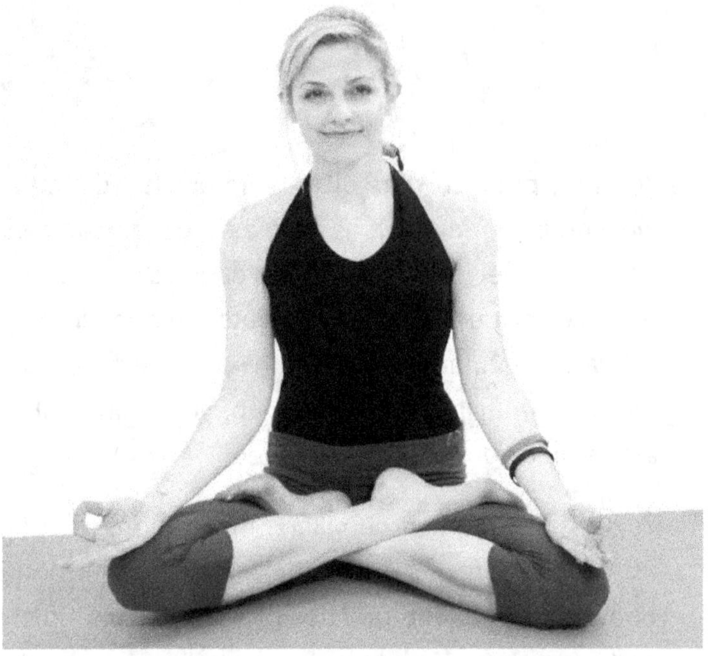

Generally, if we talk about Yoga the image of a person in the lotus posture in a state of meditation comes to mind. And yes, the truth is that PADMASANA or lotus posture is the posture used to meditate or perform pranayamas exercises because it allows us to sit "comfortably."

In this position, we must consider that the interlaced legs and the supported sitting bones must generate a firm base so that the spine is straight. The spine must be upright so that the prana flows through the spine unobstructed when doing pranayama or meditating. The hands can be placed in a particular mudra or inertly resting palms down on the knees. In this way, you close the energy circuit and manage to conserve energy in your body. It is the mother of meditation postures. If you can't cross your legs like this, place them in half Lotus (with one leg on top of the other without actually crossing).

2. Child's pose (Balasana)

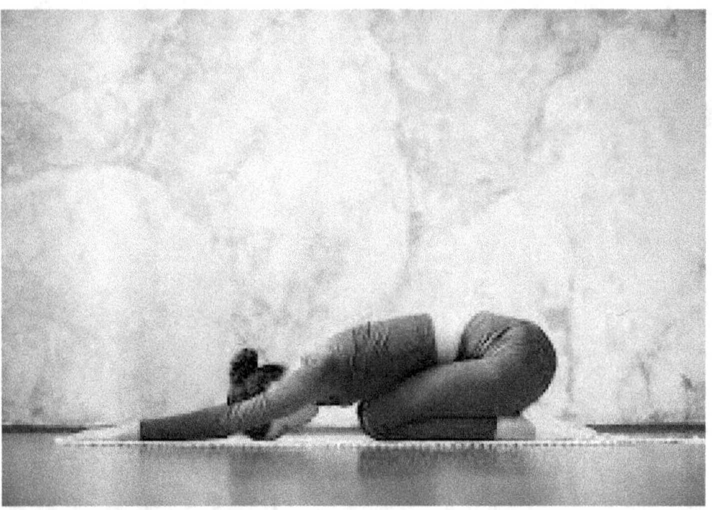

The child's pose is a submission pose. Starting from a kneeling position, with the balls of your feet touching and your knees at shoulder height, lower your waist to your ankles as you extend your arms forward, onto the ground, and lower your forehead toward the ground as well. Close your eyes and rest your forehead on the floor. Breathe in a way that is most comfortable for you.

To assume this pose, sit on your heels, spread your knees, and relax. You will notice it in the muscles of the legs and back. You will also oxygenate the brain. There is no wrong way to do the child's pose. However, if you have tight thighs, it may be helpful to place a blanket or pillow between the thighs and ankles and something to rest your forehead on.

3. Downward Facing Dog (Adho Mukha Svanasana)

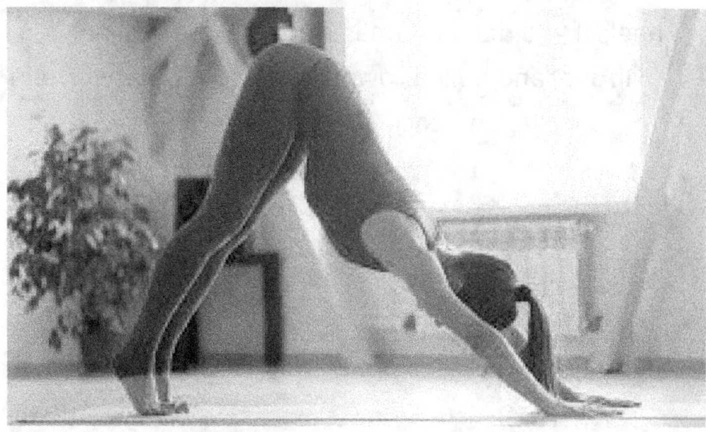

This pose opens the back of the legs, eases the spine's decompression, and allows oxygenated blood to move from the heart to the head. Start with the mountain pose. Bend following the apex of your waist and exhale as you lower your torso, keeping your spine as straight as possible. Let your head hang under its weight and relax your jaw. Keep your feet hip-width apart if you are a beginner or your feet together if you are an intermediate or advanced student.

The benefits of this asana that are essential in every yoga routine are that it tones all the back muscles of the legs and stretches the arms and spine. If you can't get your heels to touch the ground at first, don't force yourself, little by little. Keeping your spine strong is more important than keeping your legs straight. Bend your knees as much as necessary to keep your back straight and your chest in contact with your thighs.

It is more important to keep your back straight than your legs. You shouldn't hesitate to bend your knees or lift your heels if you need to. Imagine you are a fish, hooked by your tailbone, and pulled towards the boat. This will help you lift your hips up and back.

4. Tree (Vrksasana)

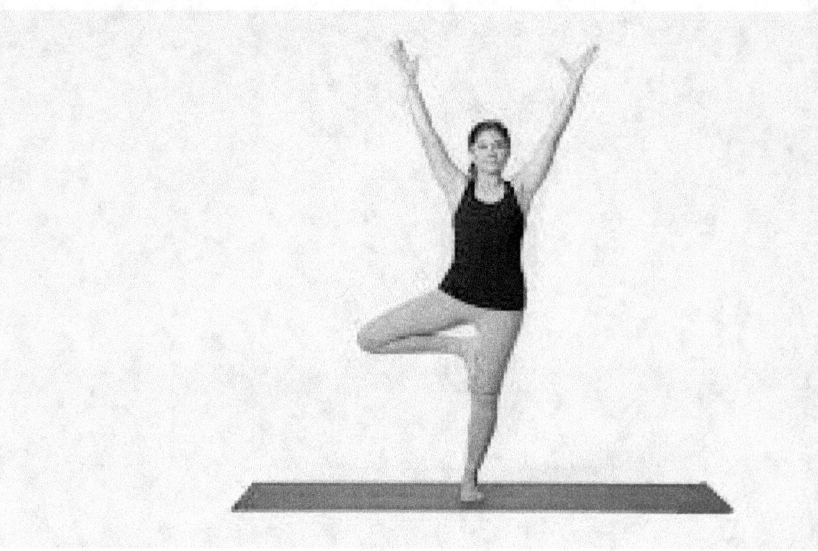

To assume this yoga pose, sand on the mat, with your hands on your waist and your elbows back. Turn your right foot and bring it up the other legs as far as you can. The right leg will be bent. Now fix your gaze on a point that you find at the level of your eyes. Stretch your arms with your palms up. Raise your arms above your head. You can join the palms of your hands. It is time to imagine that you are a tree. Raise your arms above your head. You can join the palms of your hands. It is time to imagine that you are a tree.

This pose is simple and super beneficial; what more could you ask for? Stand on one foot (put your sole on the thigh or calf) and bring your hands to your chest, ready! The key to balance is to fix your gaze on a fixed point. But it's a yogi secret. Benefits: Improves the ability to concentrate and increases energy.

5. ARADO (HALASANA)

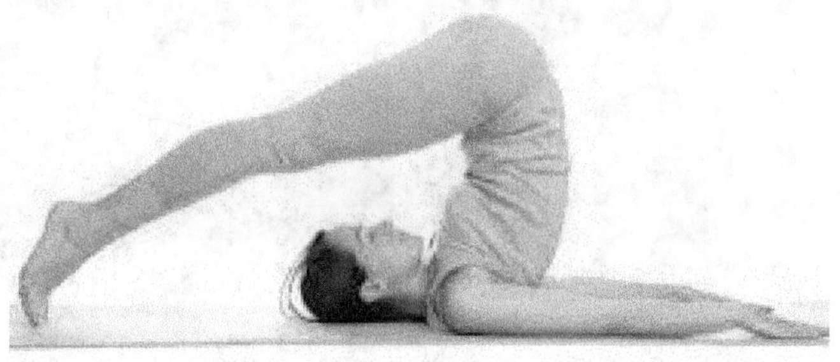

It seems complicated, but you just have to look at how the pose is done as if nothing happened. Not only will you get a photo as original as this one, but you will also stimulate digestion (constipated, this is your position). It also relieves headaches.

6. Upward facing dog (URDHVA MUKHA SVANASANA)

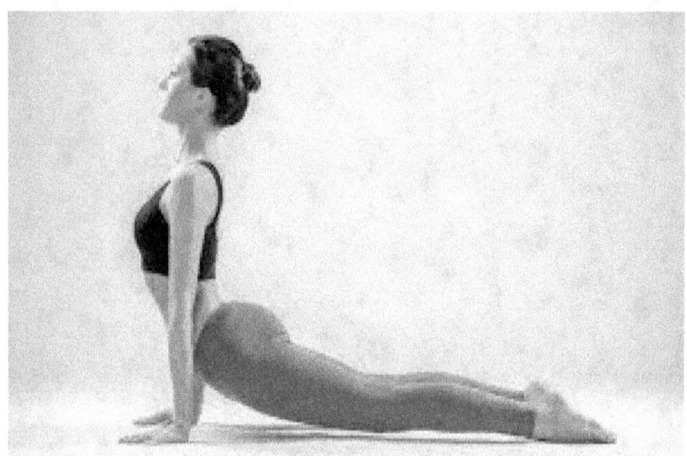

Our yogi says it can be dangerous to assume that an upward dog is a beginner's pose. It is an intermediate to advanced position since it involves a deep incline that requires a lot of force. Beginners should start with the half cobra and work their way up to the upward dog.

From a plank position, with your feet hip-width apart and your arms spread under your shoulders, exhale and use your arms to slowly lower your body until your elbows are at a 90-degree angle. Use the balls of your feet to lean your body forward, then turn your feet so that your instep rests flat on the ground. As you inhale, use your elbows to lift your entire torso, knees, and thighs off the ground. The hands and feet should be the only parts of the body in contact with the ground. Look up slightly, past the tip of your nose. Get out of the position as you exhale.

Students throw themselves into this position before their back is ready for it. It shows well when his shoulders are high and at the level of the ears. Beginners should start with the cobra pose, which is closest to the ground. The cobra barely carries weight on the hands and will slowly strengthen the back.

If you are determined to dominate the upward dog, make sure you put enough downward pressure with your feet and push your chest out using your arms. Get up from the center of the heart while pulling the shoulders down the back.

In the Sun Salutation sequence, you can incorporate the Sphinx pose (Ardha Bhujangasana), the Cobra (Bhujangasana), or this one depending on how flexible your back is and how strong your arms are.

7. Mesa (Ardha Purvottanasana)

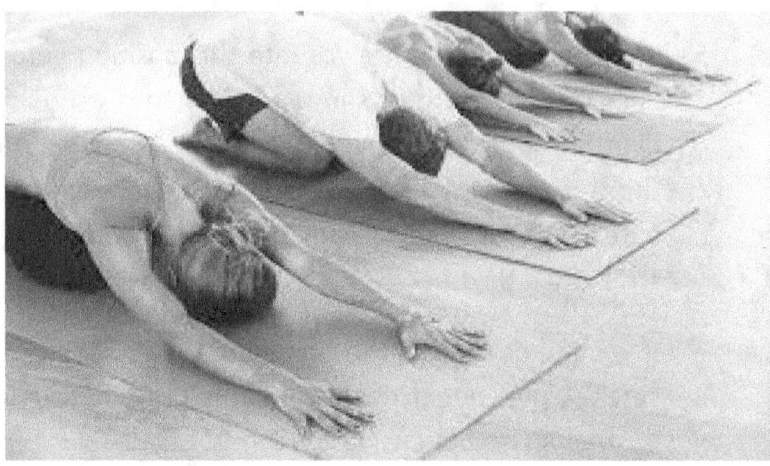

yoga also has the tremendous power of making our self-love grow and grow (to infinity and beyond). This posture strengthens the abdomen besides will also increase your self-esteem. Love yourself.

8.   Postura de Marichi (Marichyasana)

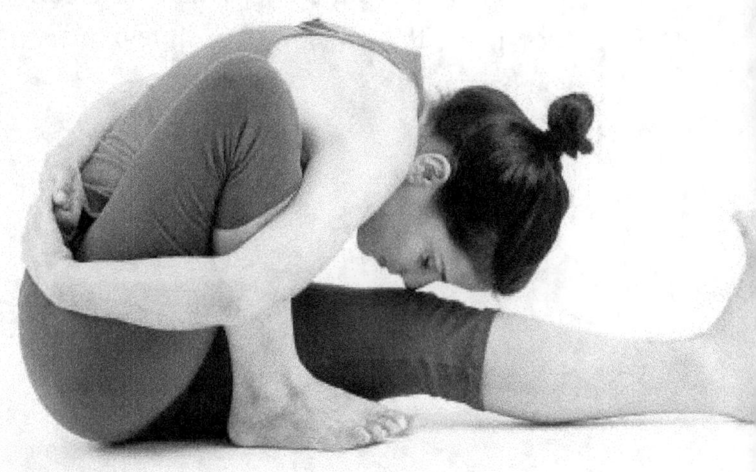

An extended leg rotation pose, dedicated to the Hindu sage
Marichi. Rotating the spine in a sitting position neutralizes
the spine. Start from a sitting position, with your butt on the
floor and both legs parallel in front of you. Fully extend your
left leg and bend your foot toward you. Bend your right
knee and cross your right foot over your extended left leg.
The left elbow pushes against the outside of the right knee;
the right hand is on the ground on the body's right side. The
right hand should be planted behind the right side of the
spine, supporting it. Look over your shoulder, or as much as

your neck allows. Repeat the pose with the opposite side of the body.

Don't turn your back. Stretch your spine by lifting your back. Make sure the backhand is helping to raise the spine. Exhale as you rotate your spine. Inhale to create space [in your torso], and the exhale will push you further into the space you have made.

9. Media cobra (Ardha Bhujangasana)

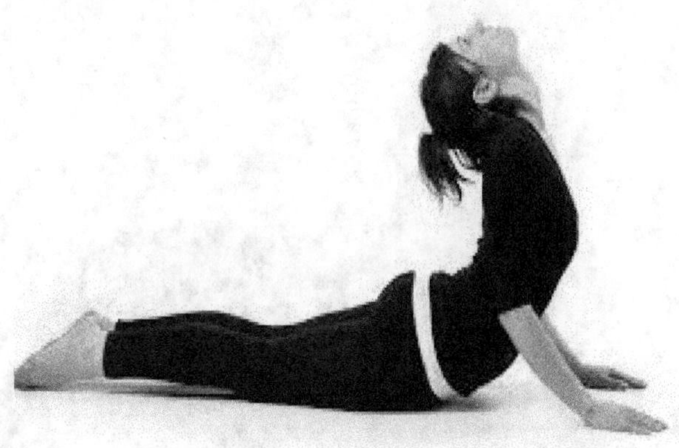

This pose is performed on the belly, with the pubic bone and insteps pressing against the ground. The feet are stretched well back and hip-width apart. The hands are placed on both sides of the rib cage, and the elbows are pulled back as if heading towards each other.

Using the strength of your lower back muscles, lift your chest and upper ribs off the ground. Inhale as you rise, breathe in a few times, and exhale as you descend.

The hands should not be in front of the shoulders, and the shoulders should not be next to the ears. To correct this, pull these back and away from your ears. Your shoulders should be at a 45-degree angle, and you should use your lower back to force -- with minimal hand thrust -- to lift your torso off the ground.

10. Triangle pose (Trikonasana)

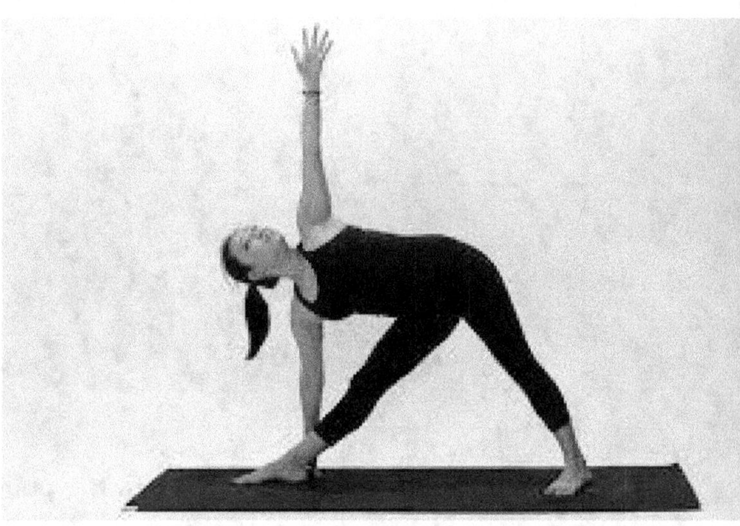

Spread your feet wide, creating a triangle from your feet to your pelvic bone. Start by turning one foot out 90 degrees and the other in 15 degrees. Stretch your arms in line with your shoulders and, as you exhale, lower your torso towards the foot that is turned out. The fingers should touch the shin; for more advanced, it should touch the ground lightly. The other arm should be stretched upward with the eyes looking at the elongated fingers' tips; keep the neck long and separated from the shoulders. The shoulders and arms should be in line.

The front hip should not stand out, and the back hip should not drop. To ensure suitable alignment, perform the pose very slowly.

11. Warrior position 1 (Virabhadrasana 1)

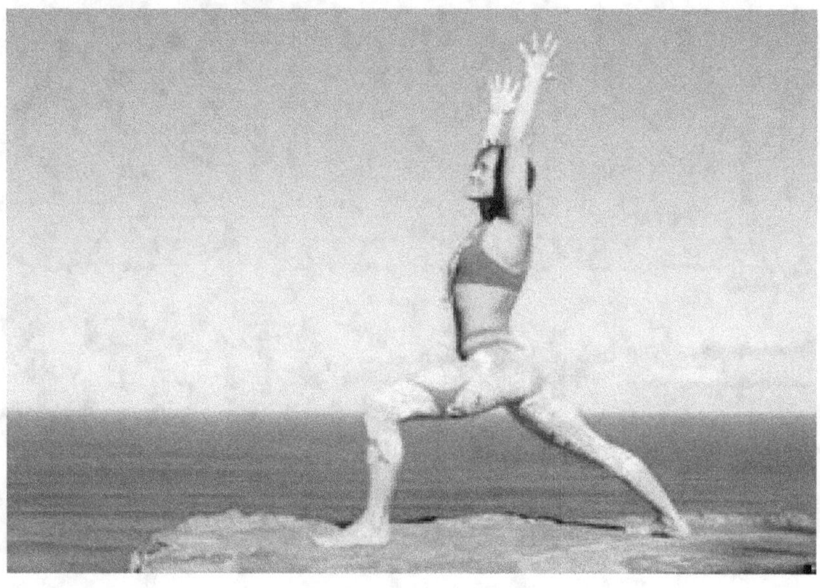

From downward dog, bring your right foot forward between your hands, turn your left heel inward, and lift your torso and arms. Inhale. The front foot's heel should be in line with the arch of the back foot, with the front of the knee directly over the ankle. Drive both hips forward, lower your tailbone, and pull your ribs inward. Repeat the pose with the opposite part of the body.

The entire waist should be facing forward, not outward, and the back foot should be approaching a 45-degree angle rather than a 90-degree angle. Imagine your hips are your two headlights. You want your headlights to face forward.

12. Warrior pose 2 (Virabhadrasana 2)

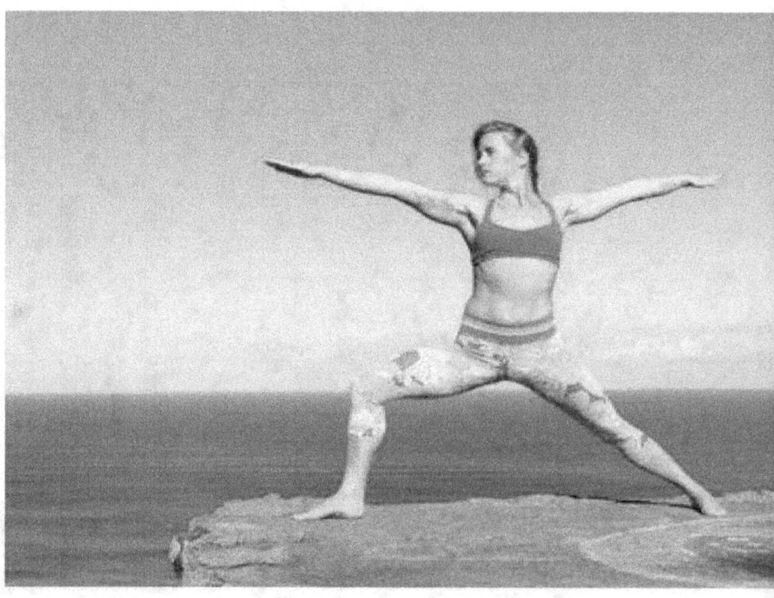

Like warrior one, but with arms stretched out in opposite directions, parallel to the ground and in line with the shoulders. Raise your arms and torso and inhale. The back foot should be at a 90-degree angle, and the front thigh should be parallel to the ground, with the knee directly over the ankle. The eyes should look over the middle finger. Repeat the pose with the opposite side of the body.

Butt and tummy should not stick out, and an arch should not form at the end of the back. Foot alignment is also a common mistake. Make sure the heel of your front foot lines up with the arch of your back foot. Imagine you are stretching your mat. To align your hips, put your hands on them to make sure you are not leaning too far over either hip.

13. Standing clamp (Uttanasana)

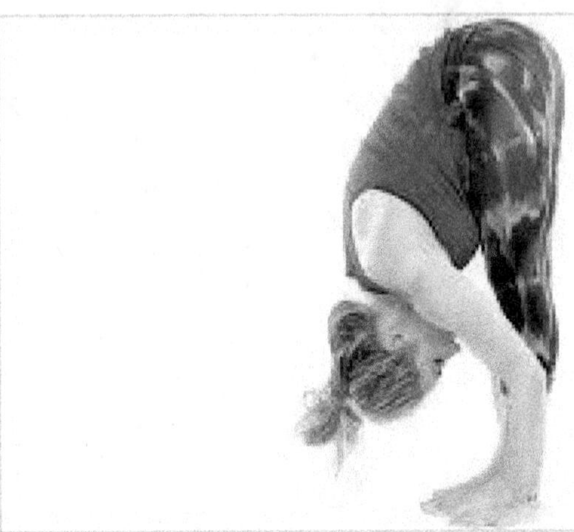

This pose opens the back of the legs, eases the spine's decompression, and allows oxygenated blood to move from the heart to the head.

Start with the mountain pose. Bend following the apex of your waist and exhale as you lower your torso, keeping your spine as straight as possible. Let your head hang under its weight and relax your jaw. Keep your feet hip-width apart if you are a beginner or your feet together if you are an intermediate or advanced student.

Keeping your spine healthy is more important than keeping your legs straight. Bend your knees as much as necessary to keep your back straight and your chest in contact with your thighs. Perseverance in Yoga is essential, and over time the back of your legs will open up with this vertical clamp. Keep your knees soft, and don't block them.

14. Chair pose (Utkatasana)

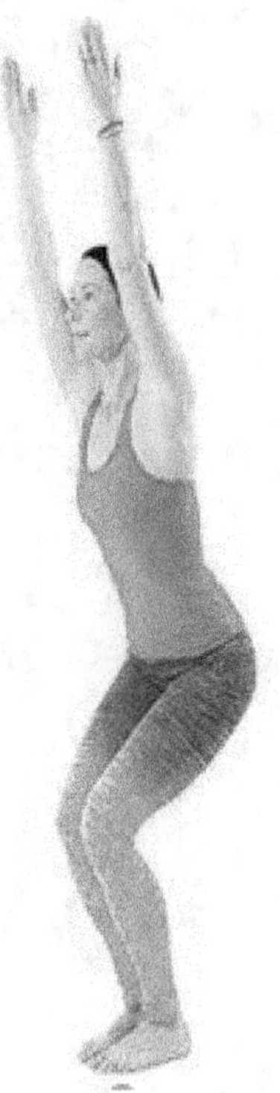

Knees bent at the ankles; thighs as parallel to the ground as possible. Your torso should be at right angles to your thighs. Bring your feet closer together to form a more advanced posture. Breathe in as you raise your hands.

The knees should not be in front of the feet. Shift more weight to your heels to pull on your knees so they don't stick out in front of your feet.

15. Mountain pose (Tadasana)

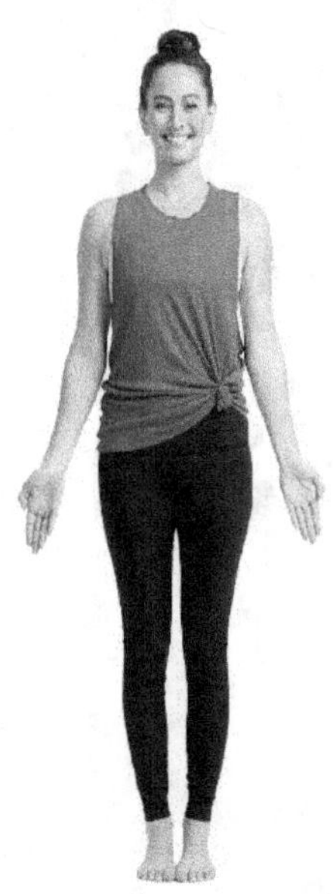

Standing, keep your spine steady with your feet parallel and the toes in contact. I look forward. Standing, honor your spine steady with your feet similar and the toes in contact. Look forward, unlike when you are usually standing, now you stand up with a purpose, feel the four corners of your feet, raise the kneecaps, distribute the weight between the legs and turn them inwards, bring the tailbone back and lift the belly button up and in. Relax your shoulders toward your lower back and bend your palms forward. Imagine you are carrying heavy stones in your hands, look straight ahead and feel the power of the mountain.

16. Bridge pose

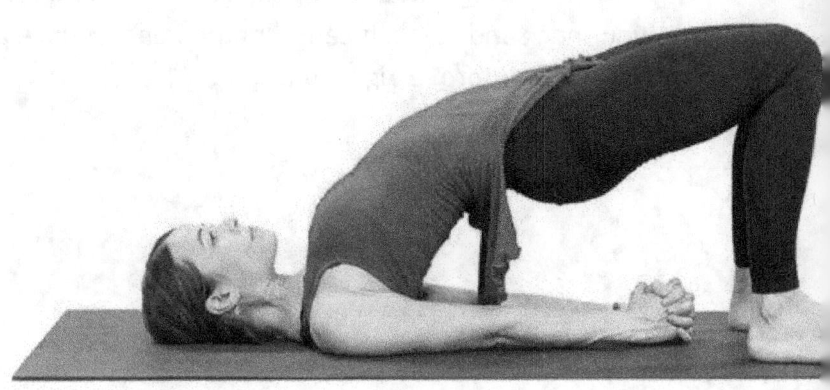

Lie faceup with knees bent, feet flat on the floor, and hands at your aspects with hands facedown. Keep your toes parallel and hip-width aside, heels stacked below knees. On an inhale, activate through the legs and the glutes. Press the ground away with your feet and lift the hips off the ground towards the sky.

If your shoulders are tight and also you want more leverage, attempt maintaining the perimeters of your yoga mat and lifting your hips. You may additionally wish to interlace your palms under your "bridge" and shimmy your shoulders beneath the chest.

When you're prepared to come back down, lift your heels up and slowly lower your hips lower back to the floor, one vertebra at a time. To keep your knees from bowing out to the side, place a block between the upper thighs. Squeeze it tight as you lift up into Bridge Pose.

This energizing backbend opens your chest and stretches your neck and spine. It can calm the mind, reduce anxiety, and assist improve digestion.

17. Seated Forward Fold

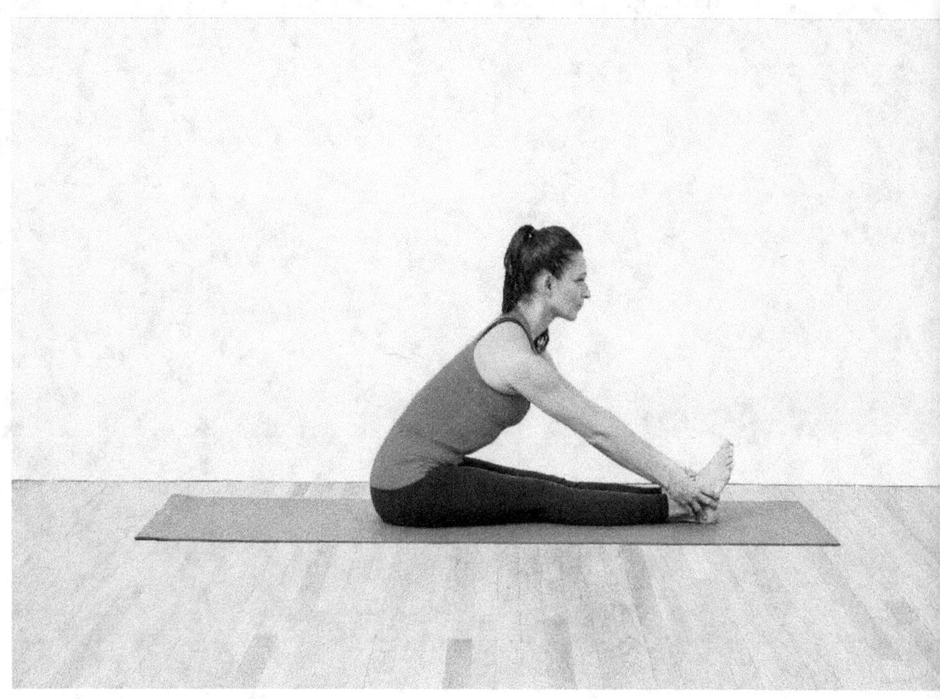

Sit and straighten your legs out in front of you, grounding your thighs into the floor. Hinge on the hips to elongate your torso over your thighs. Grab keep of the outer edges of your feet.

If your hamstrings are tight, snatch a strap and loop it in the back of your ft. Use the leverage to bring your torso closer to your thighs. You also can sit down on the edge of a blanket to help you fold ahead.

This experience-right fold elongates the again of your body, lengthens your spine, and stretches your hamstrings.

18. Corpse Pose (Savasana)

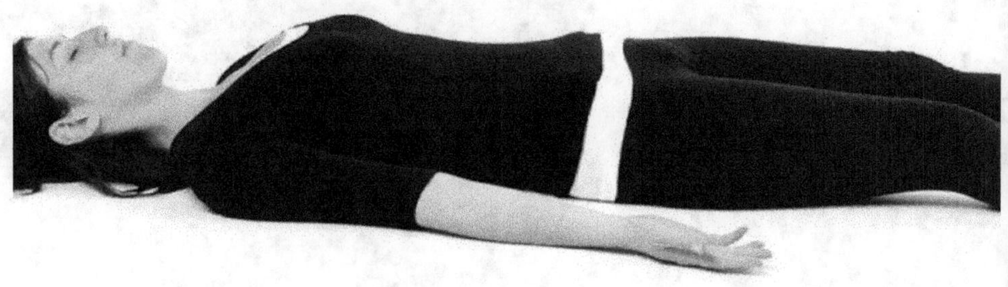

Lie faceup, bringing your legs to the outer edges of your
mat, like a starfish. Splay your feet out to the sides. Place
arms along sides, palms facing up. Close your eyes and
relax. it's as simple as it sounds. Every yoga class includes
Savasana, which relaxes the whole body and gives you
space to absorb the benefits of the practice.

19. Plank pose (Kumbhakasana)

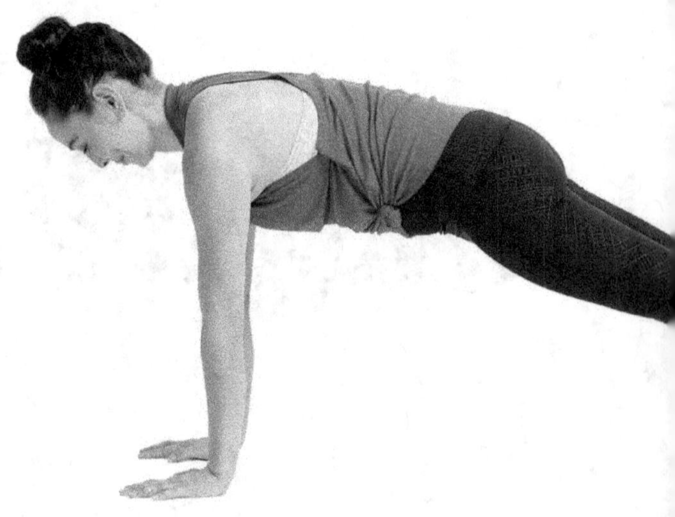

Start in Downward-Facing Dog. Shift forward so your
shoulders are stacked over your wrists. Draw your navel in
toward your spine and keep your hips from dropping.
Reach heels back as you lengthen the crown of your head
forward. Ground down into hands, pushing the floor away
beneath you. Lengthen through the arms and broaden
your chest. Come down to your knees if the pose is too
intense. It is Considered one of the best moves for core
strength, plank pose strengthens your abdominals and
promotes stability.

20. Four Limbed staff pose

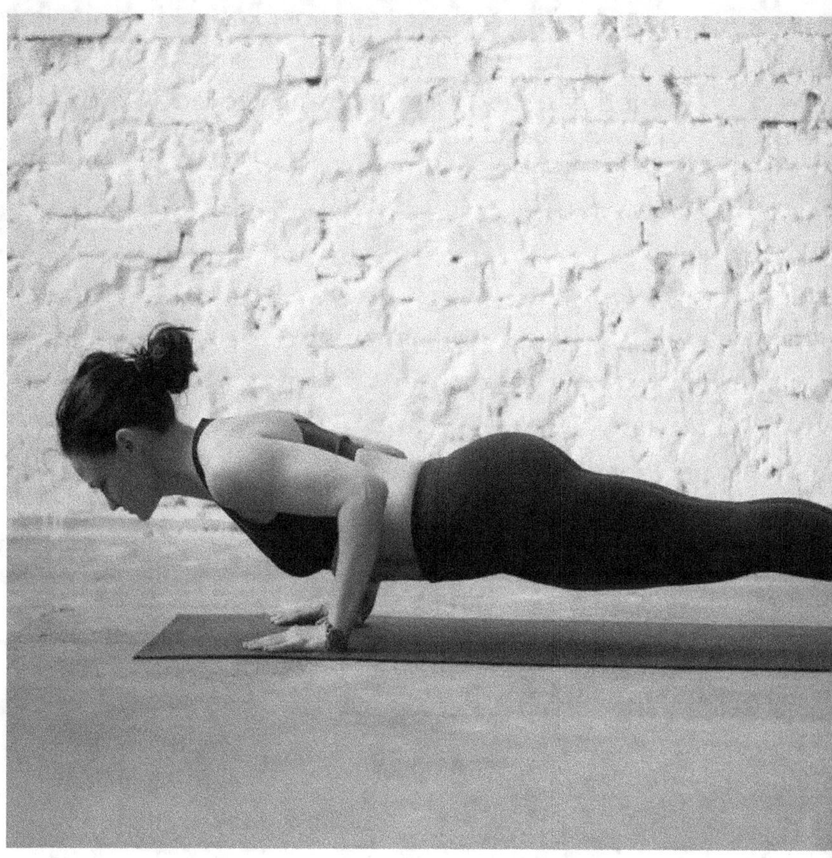

From Plank Pose, shift forward onto your tippy toes.
Ground through your palms and broaden across the chest.
Take an inhale.

On an exhale, bend your elbows to a 90-degree angle.
Keep your thighs lifted toward the ceiling. Imagine
stretching your tailbone toward your heels as you lengthen

through the spine. Hold your elbows in line with the torso. Gaze forward.

To come out of the pose, release your knees to the ground. You can also keep your knees lifted and lower down onto your stomach for an extra ab challenge. Another option is to lift up and back to a Downward-Facing Dog and relax.

MENTAL AND PSYCHOLOGICAL BENEFITS OF YOGA

The mental benefits of Yoga are unquestionable; this is a practice originally from India, which is more than 5000 years old. It is carried out by performing meditation postures, breathing, mantras, rituals, among others. In its origins, it was practiced to increase biological conservation, achieve a balance in the mind and emotions, and obtain knowledge regarding topics of philosophy such as the reason for existence, suffering, and the way to be happy inside.

Yoga is a physical and mental ancient practice expanding worldwide because of its benefits, mental stability, and guarantees a firm body and benevolent spirit. It is an old craftsmanship that has broadly demonstrated that it can improve our personal satisfaction, on an actual level as well as on a psychological and profound level. Yoga accomplishes the integration of development with the breath until these stops to be two separate elements and become one.

1. Reduce stress

The lifestyle of Western societies and the general world populace can lead many people to stress, causing psychological health problems such as depression, anxiety, etc.

Cortisol is necessary for the body as it regulates and mobilizes energy in stressful situations. Still, if we have too much or increases in cases that we do not need, it produces many side effects. By practicing Yoga can lower the levels of this hormone, and therefore reduce stress. It makes us more resistant to stress and helps us manage anxiety and clearing the mind, and bringing attention to the present moment by making the vision clearer.

Yoga, specifically Astanga yoga, is ideal for reducing stress, learning self-control, and even overcoming addictions. This modality is based solely on meditation.

2.   Increases the quality of sleep and helps you sleep better.

To achieve a peaceful rest, serotonin is also involved in controlling stress and body temperature. The practice of Yoga increases serotonin levels, so it helps you sleep better. With the approach of Yoga, you calm your mind and fill it with peace. This is very effective for those who have problems falling asleep, so it will be much simpler to sleep. Your sleep hours will be of better quality; they are valuable, as you can see the mental benefits of Yoga Improves mood.

Serotonin (5-HT) is a synapse that is gotten from an amino corrosive called tryptophan. It sends messages within the brain and through the sensory system and partakes in numerous cycles, for example, regulating mind-set or craving. One of its main assignments is to increase the creation of melatonin, a chemical that controls rest cycles. To accomplish a quiet rest, serotonin is additionally involved in controlling pressure and body temperature. The act of Yoga increases serotonin levels, so it causes you rest better.

3.   Extends life and prevents degenerative diseases

Researchers have shown that Yoga meditation increases telomeres' size, structures located at the ends of chromosomes, and are directly related to aging, the development of specific pathologies, and even premature death.

There seems to be a positive correlation between healthy and large telomeres, increased longevity, the prevention of degenerative diseases, and people's health. Doing Yoga for just 15 minutes a day is enough to produce biochemical changes in the brain and neurons.

4. Improves concentration

Yoga practitioners improve concentration, coordination, reaction time, memory, learning, and show a more remarkable ability to solve problems. 20 minutes of Yoga a day is more beneficial on a cognitive level than a session of intense physical activity. A meditative and mindful yoga practice calms the mind and makes it sharper, making us emotionally and mentally stable and robust. However, it is recommended that Yoga supplemented with a regular meditation practice.

5. Improves the relationship and sexual relations

Yoga can result in better sex because it will help your flexibility and strengthen your pelvic muscles. There are also suggestions that Yoga treats premature ejaculation and improve sexual satisfaction. The reduction of stress thanks to the practice of Yoga increases libido and sexual vitality. Therefore, by improving your sex life in different ways, your relationship may also benefit.

6. It works better

If your job exhausts you, you do not like it, or you move in a very competitive work environment; Yoga helps you get out of the dilemma without changing jobs. A Hindu study that analyzes five indicators of work performance (satisfaction, commitment, results, emotional involvement, and social relationships with colleagues) has shown that the benefits of Yoga appreciated for the worker in four of the five points analyzed; only the level of commitment was exempt from its benefits.

7. In children and students, it improves academic performance and attention.

The attention to breathing and meditation that is included in the practice of Yoga makes it possible to achieve a more peaceful state of mind, removing nerves and stress from the pressure of studies and improving performance. Or what is the same, study less and learn more and faster. It is better an hour of Yoga and a white night with coffee to pass an exam, an opposition, and a job interview.

8. Increase in consciousness

People who practice Yoga attain an increase in consciousness since when practicing it, the mind is like a journey of all the memories experienced throughout life, all this product of the imagination. It also makes it possible to focus on the present and make the most of the opportunities present.

9. Practicing yoga Increases self-esteem

Practicing Yoga makes you have a good perception of yourself and makes you aware that you can get established. It makes you use your emotions as an impulse to achieve your goals; through them, if you use them, taking advantage of their positive side, you can achieve great things.

HEALTH BENEFITS OF YOGA

There are more than ten reasons why Yoga right for you. Indeed, the physical and psychological benefits of Yoga fill entire books.

Its practice becomes a potent agent of transformation that causes profound changes in our health. Its use is seen as a preventive or rehabilitative medicine because it stimulates metabolic and anabolic processes and improves energy circulation, oxygenating the body

Therefore, the following is only a summary of the reasons that should encourage you to integrate yoga into your habits. Here are health benefits of Yoga that you should know about.

1. Your strength, agility, and flexibility are enhanced.

Lots of sports make you stronger. Others can increase your agility. But very few activities will improve your strength, agility, and flexibility at the same time. Many professional athletes have overcome their injuries by increasing their range of motion through Yoga where are even sports victims of a double mastectomy who have regained full mobility after disabling surgery, thanks to Yoga all this despite many scars on their body. Nothing is as useful as Yoga repairing the body and ensuring that ligaments and connective tissue are as strong and flexible as the muscles themselves.

2. Yoga improves memory and cognitive functioning

It may seem odd that this activity, which involves breathing and stretching, increases cognitive functions, but these are the conclusions of scientific research on this subject. According to these studies, those who practice Yoga have better learning abilities, better memory, and more effortless stay focused. These benefits are attributed to meditation, which is arguably the ultimate goal of any yoga practitioner. But meditation can also help you during your studies or at work by improving your brain's functioning.

3. Yoga stabilizes weight gain

Doing Hatha Yoga or even power Yoga probably won't burn you as many calories as a HIIT cardio session. But Yoga has the advantage of stabilizing the weight by restoring the hormonal balance in the body. Yoga lowers cortisol levels as well as our nervous system's fight or flight response. As a result, you are less likely to overeat or eat to deal with negative emotions. With Yoga, we can also teach our brain to feel full more easily since we are not constantly in panic mode! Stress is known to promote obesity, and it is the cause of many illnesses! Yoga is, therefore, perfect for counteracting these symptoms.

4.   Yoga naturally reduces pain

Many studies show that Yoga is effective in reducing pain. It doesn't matter if you have fibromyalgia, arthritis, or migraines. Yoga has been proven to relieve the pain that results from all of these ailments. If you suffer from back pain, Yoga almost makes your pain go away if like millions of people. It has even been proven that meditation can sometimes be more effective in reducing pain than morphine.

5.   Yoga increases your breathing capacity

One of the other health benefits of Yoga that it is one of the few practices that use pranayama. Pranayama is a technique based on energy and breathing. Many people practice pranayama as a means of reaching high levels of consciousness. But the health benefits don't stop there. Indeed, this practice also increases the lung capacity, the vital capacity (the total quantity of air that the lungs can contain), and the capacity to slow down its heart rate (directly related to a longer life expectancy).

6.   Regulation of blood pressure

The practice of Yoga is also beneficial for people with fluctuating blood pressure. And for those with high blood pressure, Yoga even more effective than diet modifications that can improve blood pressure.

7.   Improving mental health

Yoga offers so many benefits to the mind that it is difficult to list them all in summary. Yet, among these advantages, we can refer to an overall perking up, a feeling of generally speaking prosperity, more simplicity in communicating with others, a decline in burdensome states, less animosity towards oneself as well as other people, less uneasiness, better confidence, more inspiration, and considerably more.

8.   Yoga reduces degenerative diseases

The way Yoga averts illness is impressive. When you know-how, you'll want to grab your yoga mat more than ever! Here are some of the reasons why Yoga helps you stay young and healthy for longer. Yoga: decreases glucose, sodium, reduces total white blood cell count, lowers the overall cholesterol level, lowers catecholamines, decreases VLDL cholesterol, decreases LDL cholesterol, increases cholinesterase, increases ATPase, increases hematocrit, increases HDL cholesterol, increases hemoglobin, increases lymphocyte   count,   increases   thyroxine,   increases bioavailable vitamin C, increases the total number of serum proteins, increases oxytocin, increases prolactin.

9. The parasympathetic nervous system takes over with Yoga

Is this a good thing? The two parasympathetic and sympathetic nervous systems work together to stabilize us in the face of stress. These two systems function as communicating vessels. When one goes up, the other goes down. When the sympathetic nervous system is active, it means we are on a high alert level. Either we are reacting to stress, or we are trying to minimize it.

No one wants to be permanently amorphous or, on the contrary, permanently on the alert. It is for this reason that Yoga is excellent for mental health as it helps balance both nervous systems. As a result, it helps you not to overreact to the events you are going through.

10. You can do Yoga anywhere

Perhaps the most practical health benefit of Yoga that you can do it just about anywhere! At the airport, I have practiced in yoga studios in my house, with friends, outdoors in parks and forests, on rocks, on apartment buildings' roofs. You don't need anything (except maybe a yoga mat), although it isn't essential.

FINDING YOUR BEST YOGA METHOD

When you want to start Yoga, you can quickly be overwhelmed by the number of different practices that exist. But there is an important question you need to ask yourself; What type of Yoga is right for you?

Originally from India, Yoga takes its name from an ancient Sanskrit term meaning "to unite. " It is the union of mind, body, and soul, and the return to inner peace.

Traditionally, the desired effect has been to sit longer during meditation, calm the mind, and free yourself from the ego. The physical dimension of Yoga aims to find an anchoring, a rooting, an awareness, an intelligent alignment, and bodily mobility whose sources are strength, balance, and the absence of judgment. Yoga is a balance between mind and body, which we find thanks to the breath, which serves as our guide. There are different types of Yoga and practice over time will help you choose the right one for you. Choosing the best method for your yoga practice depends on your psychological and physical needs.

1. Hatha Yoga

In Sanskrit, "Hatha" means "strength", "perseverance", or even "tenacity". It can be broken down into two words:

"ha," which means "sun," and "tha," which means "moon." Originally, hatha yoga practice focused on mastery of the physical body serving to prepare for spiritual practice. It controls the physical body to stop the mind's flow of thoughts and reconnect with oneself.

The practice includes yoga postures (asanas), breathing exercises (pranayama), meditation, and work of subtle energies called Kundalini (kriyas). Many Yoga styles today derive from Hatha Yoga, such as Vinyasa, Iyengar, and ASHTANGA.

The point of Yoga to reconnect with yourself is to listen to the needs of the body. Please start with the poses you like and feel good about, and learn to do them correctly. This will help you develop a love of Yoga and, then add the postures you dread.

Try to practice a little bit each day, even if it's only for 15 or 20 minutes. Some days you may want to devote yourself to revitalizing postures to rebalance your nervous system. At first, don't try to have perfect posture at all costs; start with 5-10-minute sessions with simple movements, tapping into your breathing. If you are exhausted, rest in the Viparita Karani pose: lie on the floor, slide a bolster or pillows under your hips, and rest your legs against a wall. After five minutes in this position, you may have regained the energy needed for a 15-20-minute practice. But don't forget to slow down and lengthen your breaths.

I recommend that you find a teacher you like, and a course that focuses on alignment, movement, and breathing. Yoga is for everyone, but not everyone likes the same style! Try out different lessons and find a teacher and style that you like.

2. Restorative Yoga

Restorative Yoga emerges from BKS Iyengar pioneered work, who developed it in the 20th century to work with people with chronic illnesses that prevented them from engaging in more dynamic physical practice. Combined with active practice, restorative Yoga provides a balancing effect that facilitates conscious relaxation and tranquility of the mind -- one of the traditional goals of Yoga like other reflective or therapeutic approaches, restorative Yoga essentially consists of lying postures on the back. The body is often supported by props, such as a bolster, cushions, blankets, or bricks that hold the body in a position to promote relaxation. Staying for a long time in these assisted postures makes it possible to soothe chronic muscular tensions, support the natural ease of the body, and enjoy a moment of comfort by being supported by accessories.

The goal is to calm the nervous system. To reach the parasympathetic system -- that of relaxation, it is essential to use natural breathing. In a one-hour session, you may only do four poses before ending in meditation. The pace is as slow and calm as it gets, and the practice is done in a room with dim lighting. The atmosphere must be comforting.

The comfort and instructions of restorative practice naturally encourage us to calm down, turn our attention inward, and become aware of the nuances of breathing and the deep layers of being. To feel the full benefits of restorative Yoga chronic stress, it takes time -- time for your nervous system to react, to rebalance, and for that sense of space and tranquility to become the new normal.

3. Kundalini yoga

Kundalini yoga helps develop self-confidence, connections, and relationships. The practice of Yoga very beneficial against loneliness and allows you to find faith in yourself. By taking classes regularly, you join an international community and tribe. When Yoga becomes such a big part of your life, you can then train yourself to become a teacher, change your life, and the lives of others.

Dynamic Kundalini yoga includes a lot of chanting, breathing work and is always guided by an intention defined at the beginning of the course. The teacher chooses a theme for the sequence; then, each student can experience it in their way by becoming aware of what we are working on energetically through postures, breathing, and meditation.

NOTE: After you have reviewed the types of Yoga, it is time to know how to choose. Although we have included some indications in the descriptions, you may still be wondering which modality is the most suitable for you.

You want to start this practice will have a lot to do with the chosen modality. The slower and more leisurely Yoga types are ideal for beginners and those looking for a relaxation method. In contrast, the more physical ones are ideal for those who want to do light exercise and improve their physical health.

It would be best if you also kept in mind that each instructor will have their methods, so it is essential to find a center and teacher to feel comfortable. Studies have shown that yoga practitioners who have been doing this exercise the longest are the ones who most claim to notice its benefits. For this reason, it is essential not to give up on the first try. Yoga is a continuous improvement process and takes practice and time, so you cannot pretend to do everything correctly from the beginning.

Unfortunately, social media tends to present Yoga with a limited view of the body. But this is not the reality of yoga centers. There are people of all genders, sizes, and shapes practicing Yoga and a diverse and inclusive audience. Students are between 10 and 85 years old; they wear whatever clothes they feel comfortable with, whether tight leggings or lose tracksuits.

If you are new to Yoga, it's recommended that you point it out to your teacher, and don't push yourself to the point of pain. All teachers are different, and while you like a teacher's lesson, you might not like another teacher's lesson. So, try different styles and teachings to find what works for you -- your practice may follow you for the rest of your life.

HOW TO MAINTAIN RISK-FREE YOGA

you dream of taking up Yoga but something in you is scared by this discipline? Won't you get too perched from sitting in the Lotus every week? Isn't this a practice where you get easily injured by trying to gain flexibility?

Rest assured, Yoga is a discipline accessible to all ages and all audiences. Nevertheless, it is true, the drifts exist, and the risk of injury should not be ignored. So, what to do? How to reduce the dangers of Yoga. If you want to reduce the risk of injury in Yoga, it is essential to take responsibility for your practice. Whatever your teacher tells you to do or advises you, you should listen to yourself and never go too far.

Twist safely; the twists help bring flexibility to the spine, to the shoulders; they activate the blood circulation and provide a massage to the organs. All these twists "wring out" the spine. An exercise that could be scary and with good reason. Yoga twists come in many varieties; standing, sitting, inverted, or even on all fours.

The crux of all these twists is to start with a stretched spine, growing yourself. Often done too quickly, the movement must be precise and following the breathing. If the spine is not extended, you will find yourself in a tight position, which will lead to pinching at the disc level. Often, this imperfect position is not pleasant, making you feel uncomfortable.

Move your pelvis so as not to end up like a banana. Shifting the pelvis will keep the column vertical. What about breathing? It is crucial to always breathe during the effort, so you breathe to lower the legs slowly, placing the opposite arm on the ground to keep the shoulders open. The head and the gaze are directed in the opposite direction of the legs to continue the twisting, stretching at the cervical muscles' level.

Above all, do not rush. The abdominal and the exhalation will provide security to the back muscles. Therefore, by blowing, by emptying the belly, that the legs will go up slowly, the bust tightening at the level of the ribs; you will therefore use the abdominal to go up: the work is complete.

Be careful to keep in mind that Yoga is not a competitive activity, and even if the feeling of stretching, of well-being, is the goal, the pain has no place at all. The ideal is to have a professional guide to start with a good foundation and avoid injuries. So do not exceed the limits of your body.

SUMMARY

Yoga has two primary meanings: union and methods to reach this union and is a discipline and philosophy of life simultaneously that allows the collaboration of our body with our mind to achieve harmony, both on the physical, mental and spiritual plane.

Yoga is believed to be over 5000 years old, according to information from the oldest texts of humanity, the Vedas. The practice of Yoga and its culture was passed from teacher to disciple in a verbal way, and it was said that it was by word of mouth; later on, they began to be transcribed until today. The Yoga practitioner sets his own goals, becoming an experience by himself.

We live in a society of stress, nerves, and tensions. We cannot forget the pressures; this at the work and family level makes people increasingly consider looking for alternatives to download and alleviate their ailments. People seek and find in Yoga relaxation, rest, and balance while developing the mind and concentrating. There is also an essential work that cannot be forgotten, which is personal growth that helps us know ourselves. But the most important thing of all is that each person, each Yoga practitioner sets their own goals, becoming an experience by itself. There are many yoga poses and styles; choosing one should not be a problem. Identify your need to practice Yoga and find the method that meets your need; an easily adaptable approach. You do not need hours to go through these yoga activities; you only need 5 to 15 minutes each day to clear your mind and increase your concentration.